Praise for the Film
"AM I NORMAL?"

Winner of 15 prestigious film awards, AM I NORMAL? poses the questions all teenagers ask about their bodies, their sexuality, and their social lives, through the experience of three adolescent boys.

Using a humorous approach. AM I NORMAL? now followed by the female sequel DEAR DIARY—covers the sensitive subjects of body development, penis size, wet dreams, masturbation, orgasm, and peer pressure.

D0899341

Other Avon Flare Books by
Jeanne Betancourt

DEAR DIARY

AM I
NORMAL?
JEANNE BETANCOURT

Illustrations by
JEANNE BETANCOURT

Based on the film by
DEBRA FRANCO and DAVID SHEPARD

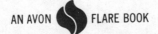

AN AVON FLARE BOOK

AM I NORMAL? is an original publication of Avon Books.
This work has never before appeared in book form.

AVON BOOKS
A division of
The Hearst Corporation
959 Eighth Avenue
New York, New York 10019

Library of Congress Cataloging in Publication Data

Betancourt, Jeanne.
  Am I normal?

  (An Avon/Flare book)
  "Based on the film by Debra Franco and David
Shepard."
  Summary: Thirteen-year-old Jimmy wonders about the
changes taking place in his body, but when he has
difficulty finding anyone to discuss them with, he pays
a visit to the library.
  1. Sex instruction for boys.   2. Puberty—Juvenile
literature.   [1. Sex instruction for boys.   2. Puberty.]
I. Am I normal?   (Motion picture)   II. Title.
HQ41.B47   1983   613.9'53   82-16282
ISBN 0-380-82040-4

First Flare Printing, February, 1983

Thanks to Rosalie Williams, educational consultant to this book, for her expertise and support.

Special thanks to Lee Minoff, Charlotte Sheedy, Jean Feiwel, and Sheldon Winicour for their invaluable assistance.

And, of course, all our love to Joel, David, and Jon.

In memory of my son

The photographs in this book are derived from the original motion picture AM I NORMAL? The Director of Photography was Nancy Schreiber. Art direction by Karla Clement.

CAST

JIMMY	Joel Doolin
TONY	David Carr
BARRY	Jon Perrigo
SUSIE	Jennifer Adelson
DAD	Downing Cless*
NURSE	Anne Lucas
ZOOKEEPER	Edward Sullivan
CRYSTAL	Crystal Sylvester
ALSO APPEARING:	Karla Clement, Ronald Coles, Jeanne Jordan, Jonathan Leinbach, Sarah McGillis, Chris Penta, Ray Romero, George Stevens, John Treworgy, Mary Whitfield

*Jerry Gershman played Dad in the film.

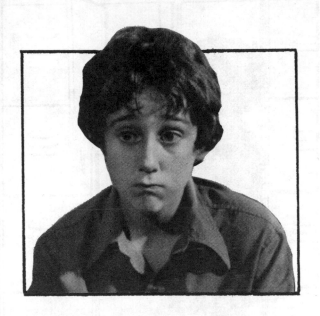

My name is Jimmy. I'm thirteen years old. I'm a pretty good kid. Yeah, without bragging, I'd say I'm a nice enough, smart enough, cool enough guy.

In fact, I used to think I was a real *normal* guy, leading a real normal life. Whole weeks would go by when the worst thing that happened to me was forgetting my history homework or getting a flat tire on my bike or not being picked right away in a choose-up game.

I usually hang out with my two best friends— Tony and Barry.

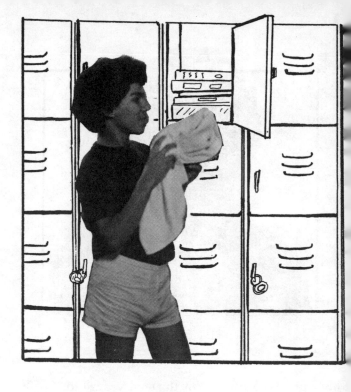

We just finished gym. The guy at the locker—that's Barry.

He's real smart and believes in homework. I bet he does it twice, just to be sure he's got it right. Barry's quieter than me, but when he says something you can be sure it's exactly what's on his mind. Barry's a doer. He belongs to practically every club in school. He's first-string on the J.V. Video Games Team.

And here's good old Tony! While Barry's rushing around to get from gym to math, Tony's taking his sweet time.

Tony's first rule of life is: "Don't rush. Be cool."

His second rule of life has to do with homework: "Don't do it. Be cool."

Tony on grades: "Grades? Who needs them? I *know* I'm great. Be cool."

Tony has grown to be the biggest guy in the whole class. He's even taller than most of the eighth-graders. Maybe that's why everyone looks up to him.

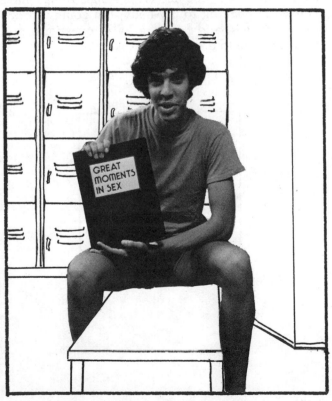

The three of us do everything together. We play three-man basketball, watch the same TV shows, laugh at the same jokes.

But I have to tell you, things haven't been going so smoothly for me lately. Strange things have started happening to my body, I'm going through these changes, and I have a lot of questions. And they all have to do with sex. Like:

Masturbation?

Erections?

Wet Dreams?

Hair?

4

I'm beginning to wonder...

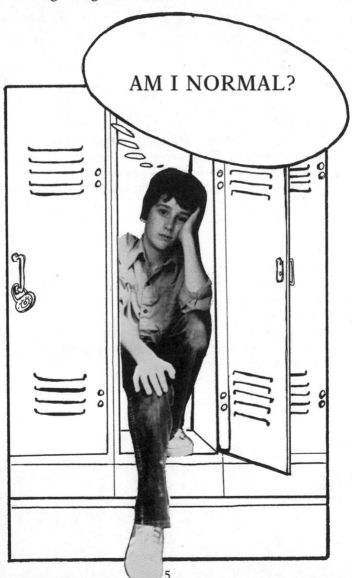

Now, I know my buddies think a lot about sex too—especially Tony. Sex is what Tony talks about *all* the time, and the only thing he *ever* reads about.

But what he tells us just makes things worse for me. He's been telling us a lot of strange stories and jokes. A guy doesn't know what to believe, which is probably one of the reasons I've been so confused lately.

Here goes Tony with another of his stories. He's reading this one from his favorite book, *Great Moments in Sex*, by Stanislaus Ripemoff. You'll see what I mean.

"Hey, hey, hey, guys," Tony shouts, as he looks around to be sure that Coach Morris isn't in the locker room. "Listen to this."

Then he reads, in his slow stop-start way: "'Jack Market of London, England, had an e-rec-tion which was two feet long. He held it there for forty-eight days, and three people sat on it before it finally snapped off.'"

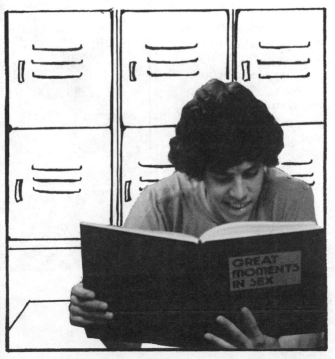

Everybody thinks about that for a few seconds. A couple of the guys snort and chuckle. I wonder, *Is it true or not?* Nah! It can't be true—or can it?

Barry must be thinking the same thing because he looks up from tying his shoelace and asks, "Is that stuff really true?"

Tony looks at me and winks. "Hey, Jimmy, it's true, isn't it?"

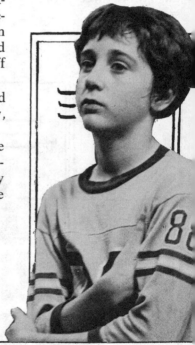

Tony says, "Of course it's true. It—ah—happened to a friend of my brother. Come on. Be cool."

I turn around. All the guys are looking at me. I have to stay cool. "Yeah, man, of course it's true," I say. But I don't really believe it.

Then I sneak out of the locker room fast before Tony comes up with another one of his stories.

* * *

The next morning I'm one of the first kids at the hall locker before home room. I notice Susie coming down the corridor. And she sees me.

Susie is in my home room and some of my classes. She's always smiling at me. Last week when we were choosing sides for a debate on nuclear energy she made sure she was on my team.

Having a girl who likes you can be real awkward. Like yesterday, Susie's friend, Teri, passed me a note in math that said, "Do you like Susie? Check one. Yes. No." I didn't know what to do, so I just ignored it.

Last year I didn't like girls. I mostly thought they were pretty silly. But this year things are different. It's hard to explain. But I can tell you this much, I feel differently about girls than I did in sixth grade. And I do like Susie.

Anyway, she comes over to my locker and stands *right next* to me.

"Hi, Jimmy. Can I read over your history notes during home room? I forgot mine."

"Sure," I tell her. "I'll bring them."

Uh-oh. What's this feeling? What's happening to me? Oh, no, not here. Not right now!

No question about it. I'm getting a whatever-you-call-it. Right. An erection, right here in the hallway.

I shove my hands in my pockets to try to hide it.

"What are you doing?" she asks in her nice way.

"Looking for my keys," I blurt out. "I can't find my keys."

Pretty clever excuse, huh? Except I think I'm beginning to blush.

"Can I help?" she asks innocently.

My heart sinks. "No, I'd rather you didn't," I say with a weak smile.

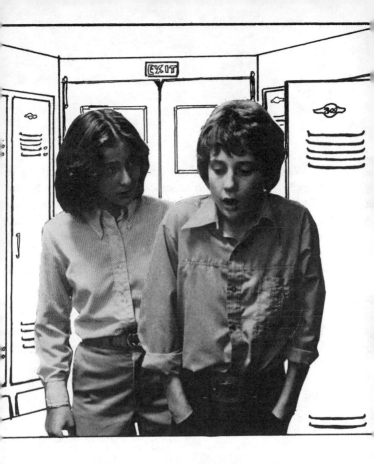

"Okay, Jimmy." She starts to go, but then turns around and asks, "By the way, would you like to go to the movies this weekend?"

"Ah—sure...I guess," I mumble.

"Great." She flashes me a smile and finally leaves.

Was that ever a close call! What's happening to me? Why did I get an erection in public and in broad daylight? I wonder if this ever happens to the other guys, or am I the only one whose body is, well, out of control?

The next day after basketball practice, Tony, Barry, and I are joshing each other about sex again, telling the usual dumb jokes. I keep wondering about the erection I had yesterday.

I look at the guys. Does it happen to them? It seems like something you should be able to ask your friends. I mean, we're always talking about sex anyway.

While I'm thinking this, I hear myself saying much too loud, "Hey, guys, I have a question."

Barry looks up from getting his books ready for class.

Tony looks up from ogling pictures of naked ladies in his magazine.

Everybody is looking at me.

You know how sometimes you know you're making a mistake while you're doing something, but you do it anyway? This was one of those times for me.

While one part of me was saying, "You dummy, don't ask them this," the other part of me was saying very loudly:

"I was wondering. See, I got a hard-on in the hall for no reason. It happened the other day during math too. Am I normal? I mean does this ever happen to you?"

DEAD SILENCE!

Everyone, including me, is looking at Tony to see what he'll do.

A slow smile starts at the corners of his mouth.

Will he answer me? Maybe it wasn't so dumb to ask after all. Maybe I'll get an answer.

Wrong!

Tony's smile turns into his snorty laugh, and then into a howl.

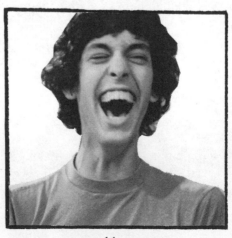

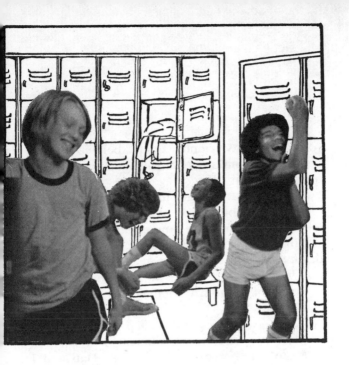

Nobody answers my question. Guys who are falling off benches, rolling all over the floor, laughing hysterically aren't too good at answering questions.

I look at my friends. I can't believe what a big deal they're making over this. I asked a reasonable question, didn't I?

I feel hurt and angry and they're laughing.

I'm also embarrassed, so embarrassed that I laugh too, so they won't see how awful I really feel.

I'm more puzzled than ever. On the way home I think over and over, *Who can I talk to? Who won't laugh at my questions? Who has some answers?*

Just as I get to my street corner it comes to me. My dad!

* * *

After supper I see my chance.

Mom's at her exercise class, so Dad and I are alone.

Dad's in the living room in his easy chair clutching the remote control for the TV. A baseball game is on—a real dull game, so I know he won't mind being interrupted.

A word about my dad.

He looks and acts like a teddy bear. He likes me and I like him.

Dad loves to do things for me. Like once when my mother said I had to finish cleaning the garage before I could play softball, my dad sneaked out and helped me so that I wouldn't be late for the practice. Not all dads would do that.

I definitely have a good dad. But I feel funny asking him about sex. It's something we've never talked about. Basketball, football, cars—yes. Sex—never.

Here goes. I sit on the edge of the chair opposite him. "Dad?"

He looks up real nice and says, "Yes, son?"—like I'm about to ask him if he wants another dish of ice cream.

I look at the floor. "Dad, can you tell me about, uh, sex?"

He zaps off the TV and swivels his rocker toward me. He looks all concerned. "What's the matter, Jim? Are you in trouble or something?"

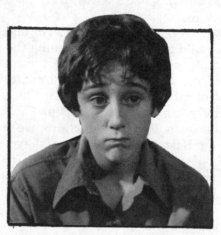

Trouble? "No, Dad, I'm not in any trouble."

I look up at him. "I'm in confusion. Nobody at school seems to know what's going on and a lot of crazy stories are going around. I thought you could..."

"Oh...I see. You want to know about...sex?"

I nod.

"That's terrific, son. Just between you and me,
right? Man to man, father to son. You know, my
father never talked to me about ... that kind of stuff.
Okay, let's see now ..."

Finally some answers! I told you he wouldn't
laugh.

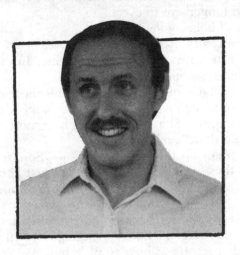

Dad leans forward and so do I. We're eye to eye,
man to man.

"Son, it's like this," says Dad, shifting in his seat.
"Men have—uh—their own baseball bats."

He frowns for a second and tries again. "No, no.
That's not it," he continues. "Um—girls have catch-
er's mitts and boys have a—well, no..."

Poor Dad's wiggling like crazy in his easy chair. He keeps glancing back at the blank TV screen. We are no longer eye to eye.

"Am I helping you, son?"

"Not really, it's just that—"

He interrupts, "Okay, let's do this, Jim. There's first base, second base, and—"

"No, Dad, I mean, what about all these changes that are going on in my body and everything?"

"Changes?" That word makes him more uncomfortable than "sex" did.

He picks up the remote control. "Son, men just know these things. That's all, they just know. It'll come to you. You'll see. Don't worry about anything. Now I'm gonna watch my game."

He zaps the set back on and swivels his rocker to face the screen. "Look at these guys, will ya? We should teach them how to play ball. We could do better than those yo-yos. What do you think?"

"Sure, Dad," I say. "I've got some homework to do."

I go to my room. I just sit there watching my white mice, R2D2 and Godzilla, running round and round on their wheels.

"*Men just know these things.*" Well, I sure don't know them. I don't feel like I know *anything*. Does that mean I'm not a man? When will I understand what's going on in my body? Shouldn't I know what's going on while it's happening?

I'm more confused than ever.

And that's how I fall asleep—confused.

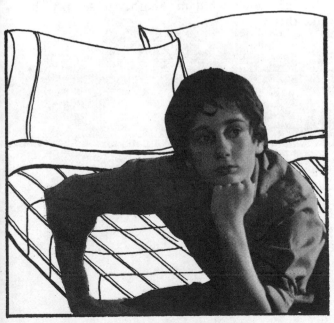

The next morning my alarm doesn't wake me up. A sticky, wet feeling in my pajamas does. At five A.M.

Have I wet my bed? No, it's too thick to be that. I remember that I was dreaming when I woke up. This must be what the guys mean by a "wet dream."

I sure don't want my mother to see my sheets like this.

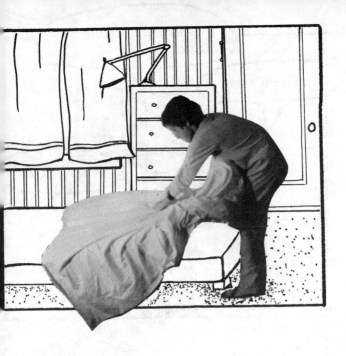

I'd better hide the evidence.

I creep down the hall.

I very carefully open the bathroom door so it doesn't creak.

It creaks.

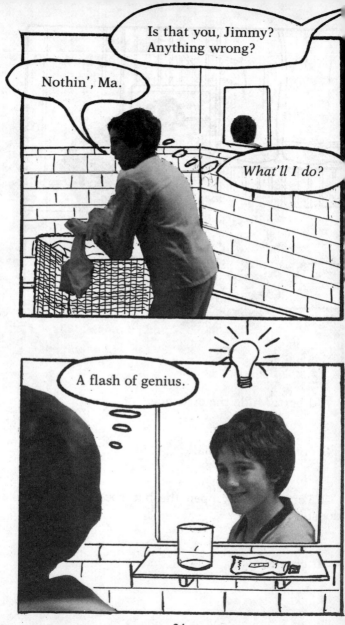

24

I pour a glass of water on the sheet as I call to my mom.

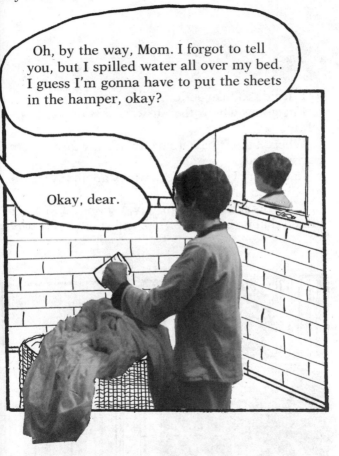

Oh, by the way, Mom. I forgot to tell you, but I spilled water all over my bed. I guess I'm gonna have to put the sheets in the hamper, okay?

Okay, dear.

I stuff the sheets in the hamper. Boy, my life is becoming more and more ridiculous.

I decide to take action.

I'm going where the answers are in black and white.

Where I don't have to deal with my father's embarrassment.

And where I don't have to worry about my friends making fun of me.

After breakfast on Saturday, I set out. I'm determined that no one, but *no one* will stand in my way.

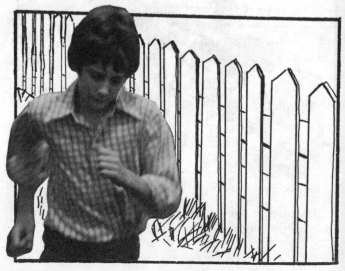

I turn the corner in front of the playground and there's Tony.

I nod hello as I run past him. I figure it this way: If I look like I'm in a hurry to run an errand or something, he won't bug me.

I'm wrong.

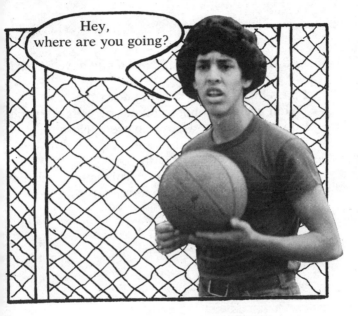

"To the library," I answer.

At least Tony won't want to come with me. Tony doesn't believe in books. He says that if God wanted us to read he wouldn't have made television.

And there's Barry, too. Can't a guy have any privacy?

I pass him without slowing down.

"What are you going to read?" he yells after me.

I don't look back when I answer, "Nothin'."

Barry is definitely the kind of guy who would love to go to the library with you.

But I don't want company. This is one research assignment I'm going to do *alone*.

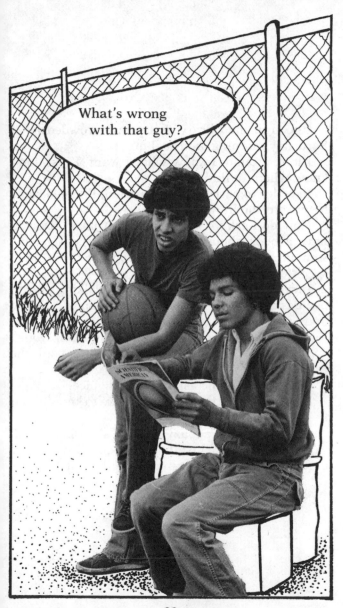

I go into the library. It's pretty crowded for a Saturday morning, and real quiet.

I look around. I know what I want, I just don't know where to find it.

In order to carry out my mission, I'll need some help from the librarian.

How do I ask for what I want? If I say, "Do you have a book about the male body," she'll get me something on body building. I've got to be more specific, but how?

I try to figure this out while I'm walking over to her desk. Maybe I should ask for a book on male body parts. No, that sounds like auto repair.

The librarian looks up at me. "Can I help you?"

I whisper, "I want a book about...about the male...penis."

"Excuse me?" she asks in a loud voice.

I try again, a little louder. "I'd like to know about the male penis, please."

I'm blushing like crazy, but she's perfectly cool. "Yes, of course, I've just the right book for you. Why don't you wait at that table and I'll get it."

I sit down and she disappears into the stacks. I can't believe it.

A few minutes later she comes back and hands me a big book. "This book might be helpful."

I open it.

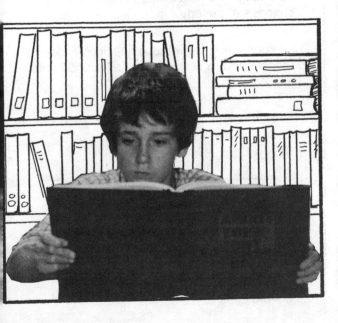

Maybe now I'll get some answers.
This is what I read:

ABOUT PUBERTY

Between the ages of eleven and fifteen, boys go through the physical, emotional and sexual changes of puberty.

Your voice will gradually become deeper (although for a while it may just sound hoarse and crackly).

Hair begins to grow on different parts of the body, including the pubic area.

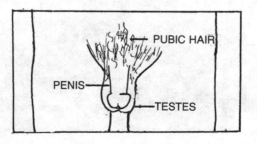

Your body may start to grow very quickly, as you begin to develop your adult size and shape.

During this time, the PENIS and TESTES gradually become larger. They also become very sensitive to sexual feelings and thoughts.

These changes may happen separately, or around the same time. Some boys will start to grow early, around eleven, and some not until much later—fifteen or sixteen.

Remember, everybody is different.

ABOUT THE PENIS

The penis is made up of spongy tissue and blood vessels.

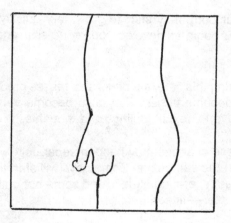

Certain thoughts or feelings or sexual activities can cause these vessels to fill with blood.

When this happens, the penis becomes hard and erect. This is called an ERECTION.

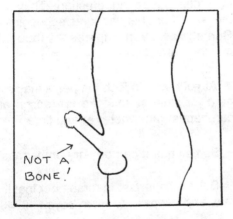

NOT A BONE!

Even though it may feel like it, an erect penis is NOT a bone. It cannot break or snap off.

Many different kinds of thoughts and feelings can cause an erection. They may be pleasant thoughts, thoughts about girls or sex. Sometimes even unpleasant thoughts can cause an erection.

At your age, in fact, the penis may even get hard for what seems like no reason at all. It can happen anywhere, at any time.

Sometimes it can be very embarrassing!

But it is important to remember that it is normal, and happens to most boys.

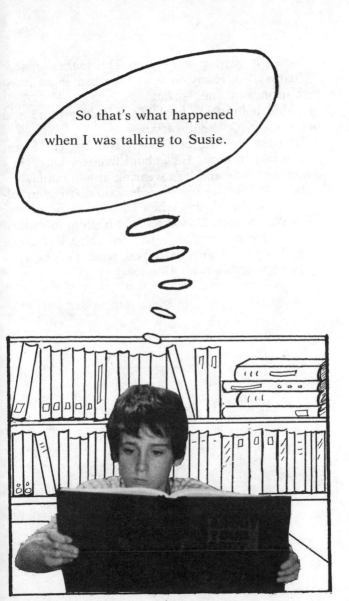

37

Now I'm getting someplace. This makes sense.

Just as I'm ready to start the chapter on masturbation, in comes—Tony!

I hide behind my book. Tony looks around and heads right for the librarian.

"Excuse me," he practically shouts. "Have you seen a boy in here? He's about five feet four. He's got brown hair and he's wearing brown pants."

What's Tony up to now? He didn't bother to follow me to the library when I was working on my Civil War report. This guy is *not* trailing me out of concern for my welfare. He must think I'm up to something and wants to find out what. He's becoming a regular Sherlock Holmes.

Tony or no Tony, I'm not giving up when I'm just starting to get some answers.

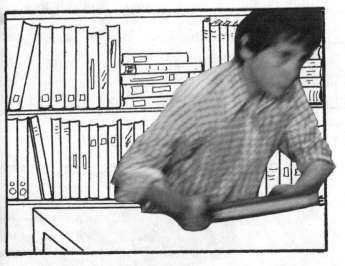

I duck into the men's room.

39

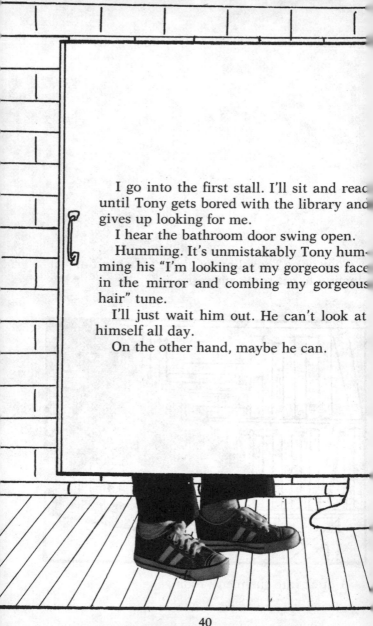

I go into the first stall. I'll sit and read until Tony gets bored with the library and gives up looking for me.

I hear the bathroom door swing open.

Humming. It's unmistakably Tony humming his "I'm looking at my gorgeous face in the mirror and combing my gorgeous hair" tune.

I'll just wait him out. He can't look at himself all day.

On the other hand, maybe he can.

"Hey, Jimmy, man, you've been in there an awful long time. What are you doing?"

How does he know I'm here? I look at the floor. My red sneakers gave me away. I should have stood on the seat. Too late now, so I answer him, real matter of fact: "I'm reading."

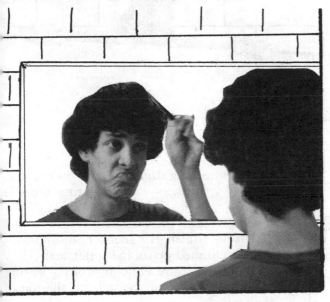

"Yeah, sure you're reading," he chuckles. "I know what you're doing in there. Feeling good, huh? Come on now, you can tell old Tony boy."

So *that's* what he thinks I'm doing. I hear him walking toward my stall. "You'd better watch out. If you do it too much, it's going to fall off. They say you can grow hair on your palms. You know—leprosy. Ever hear of that? It's true!"

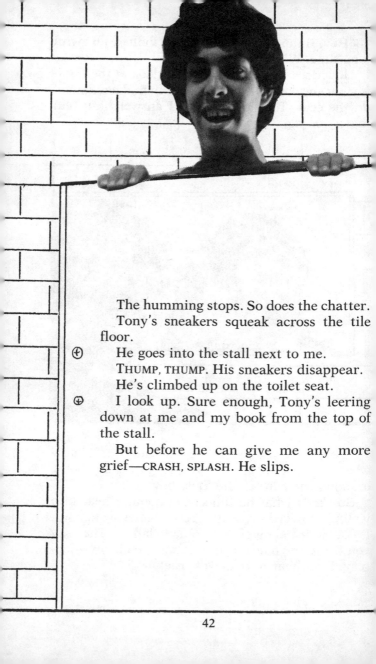

The humming stops. So does the chatter.

Tony's sneakers squeak across the tile floor.

He goes into the stall next to me.

THUMP, THUMP. His sneakers disappear.

He's climbed up on the toilet seat.

I look up. Sure enough, Tony's leering down at me and my book from the top of the stall.

But before he can give me any more grief—CRASH, SPLASH. He slips.

I laugh. The thought of Tony with one foot in the toilet bowl is pretty funny and not too cool. But good old Tony acts like nothing happened.

"Yeah, man," he calls to me. "I gotta be going. Just remember what I said, okay? Catch you later."

Instead of thinking about what Tony said, I'll just read what the library book says.

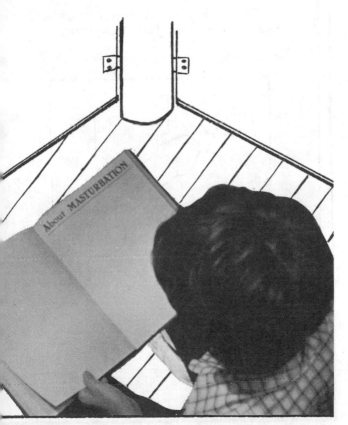

ABOUT MASTURBATION

For a male, masturbation is touching or stimulating his sexual organs, causing the penis to become erect.

Often he will masturbate until the penis spurts out the milky white fluid called SEMEN.

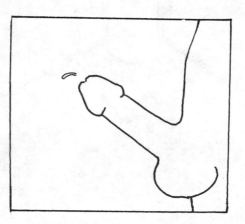

This is called an EJACULATION.

EJACULATION is often accompanied by a special intense feeling called ORGASM, after which a person feels relaxed.

It is important to remember that just because you have an erection, it isn't necessary to have an ejaculation.

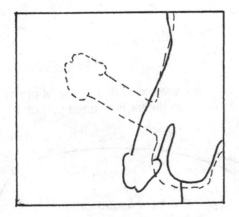

Even if you don't ejaculate, the erection will soon go away on its own.

You may have heard stories about how masturbation is harmful. (Some of the more ridiculous ones are that it can make you go crazy or have hair grow all over your body.)

That's what Tony was saying!

But we know today that it cannot physically hurt you—no matter how often you do it.

So that business about leprosy isn't true either.

Many people of all ages—men and women—masturbate.

They do it because it gives them pleasure and relaxes them. It is also a way of getting to know their bodies and feeling good about them.

Other people may not enjoy it, or find it against their principles. Masturbation is a private act and a private decision.

IT IS NORMAL IF YOU DO IT.

AND ALSO NORMAL IF YOU DON'T.

Over the rest of the weekend I think a lot about what I've read. I'm feeling pretty good, like I'm getting a handle on my problems. And some answers to my questions.

Then Monday morning I wake up to a reminder of a big question that I haven't quite gotten an answer to.

Why do I have wet dreams?

This becomes the question that bugs me the most.

As Monday moves along from history to math to science to lunch, what begins to bug me even *more* than my question is Tony.

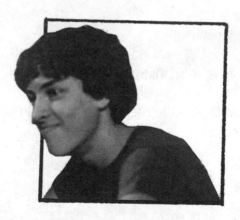

He's watching me like a hawk. And whenever I catch him looking at me he just grins real mischievously.

On our way to lunch, as we're passing Susie and her friends, Tony whispers real loud, "I'm warning you, Jimmy, hairy palms. What girl's gonna want to go out with a guy with hairy palms?"

Boy, if Tony was a foot or so shorter, he'd really be asking for trouble from me.

During English, our class is called down to the nurse's office for our annual vision test. All thirty of us line up outside Nurse Sheedy's door.

I get the bright idea that if Barry, Tony, and I are at the end of the line we'll miss most of Mr. Kane's English class.

I make sure I'm the last on line. This is very clever of me because I've decided to ask the nurse the questions I have, and I sure don't want any of the kids in my class to overhear me.

Nurse Sheedy is friendly and all smiles, but she wants to get right down to business.

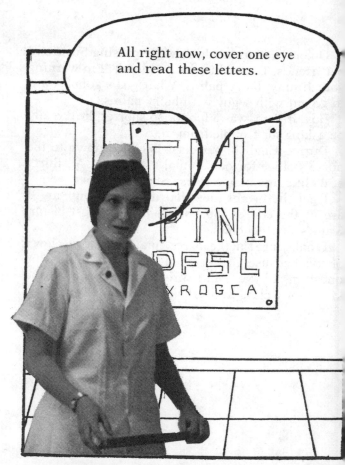

Do I dare ask her? I figure it this way, I can't let a great chance like this pass me by.

I take the plunge.

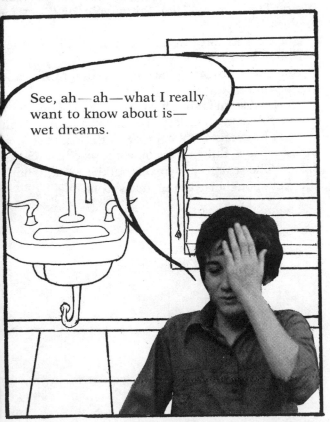

"Oh. Did you have a wet dream last night? Well it's perfectly normal for a boy your age. Let me explain it to you."

She acts as natural and calm as if I had asked her how to brush my teeth.

She pulls down a chart with a diagram— and guess what's on it?

"A wet dream is simply an EJACULATION that happens while you are asleep. When you ejaculate, this is what happens. SPERM, made in the TESTES, combines with a fluid to become the mixture called SEMEN. The SEMEN then travels out the PENIS. That's the wet spot that was on your sheets."

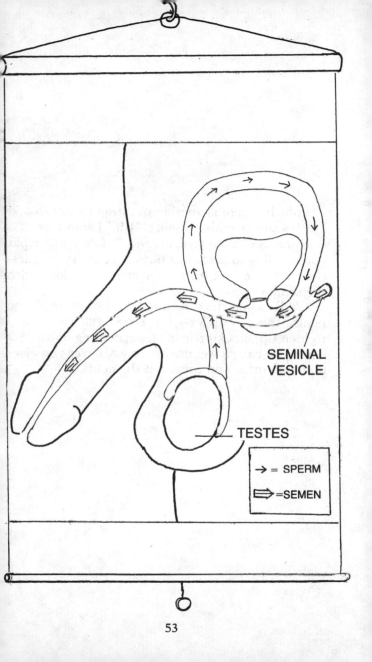

SEMINAL
VESICLE

TESTES

→ = SPERM

⇒ = SEMEN

I blush. There is another question I want to ask, but it's pretty embarrassing. "Uh," I stammer...

Nurse Sheedy interrupts me. "I know just what you're going to ask! Most boys have the same question. Why doesn't urine ever come out along with the semen?"

"Well, while the semen is traveling through the penis, these muscles—the SPHINCTER MUSCLES— tighten up, blocking urine from coming down. So when you have a wet dream, or whenever you ejaculate, no urine can come out the penis."

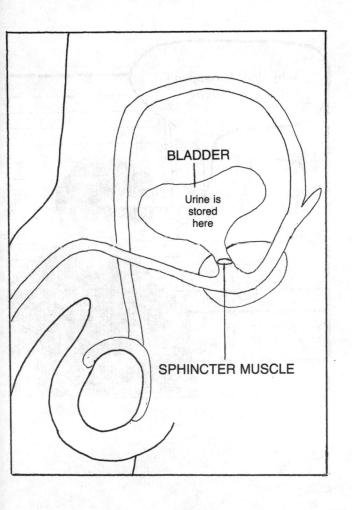

BLADDER

Urine is
stored
here

SPHINCTER MUSCLE

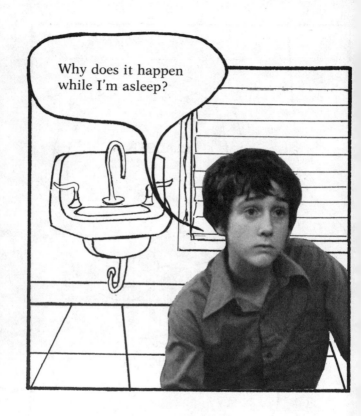

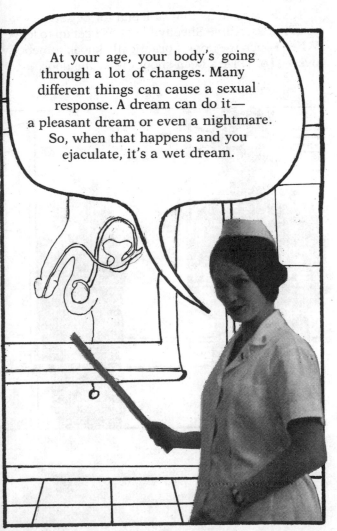

It's as simple as that? I feel a lot better.

"Thanks, Nurse Sheedy," I say as I get up to leave. When I open the door, I practically knock somebody over—Tony. He's been snooping at the door.

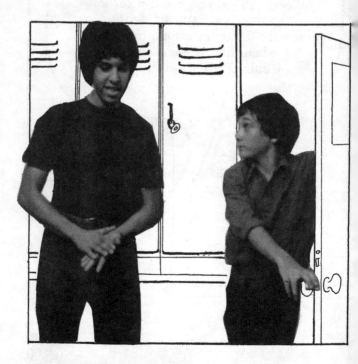

I wonder if he was listening the whole time. If he was, I figure I'm in for a lot more ribbing. But he's actually a little embarrassed.

It doesn't take him long to recover, though. "Ah, hi there, big Jim. Just thought I'd wait around for you. Protect you from the girls on the way back to class."

The rest of the week is pretty normal. Mostly because *I'm* feeling normal again.

* * *

Saturday morning the three of us head for the zoo, our usual weekend hangout.

Tony starts talking about sex, of course. "Can you imagine if that one was human? Boy, that's what I call *macho*. Take a look at the size of the thing that lion's got."

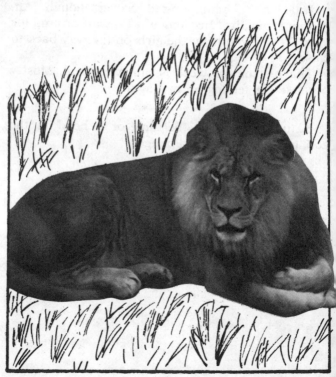

I'm not about to argue with Tony. But I wonder, *'s Tony saying that the guy with the small penis is ess of a man? And how small is small?* This is con-*using.

Barry looks as puzzled as I feel, only he's brave enough, or dumb enough, to question Tony: "I heard size doesn't make a difference."

"Don't be stupid," Tony tells him. "Of course it does. It's got to. It's only logical. Just think about it for a minute."

I duck out as Tony is telling Barry, "Anyway, you and I don't have to worry. On the other hand, little Jimmy here..."

When Tony looks around at me, I'm long gone.

I notice the zookeeper sweeping up near the mon key cages. I've seen him around the zoo a lot. He' a nice guy who knows all kinds of interesting stuf about animals. And he's always glad to share it.

I watch him for a while. When he notices me he looks up and smiles.

"What can I do for you, son?"

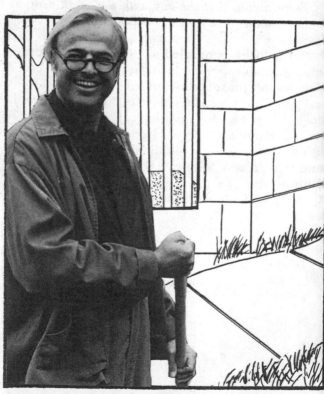

I decide this is another one of those opportunities I can't pass up. I try to swallow my embarrassment. "Well, I have this question. It's kind of a biological thing."

"Okay, shoot," he says.

For a second I try to think up a different question, like what do you feed the monkeys, or something. But my courage comes back when I open my mouth.

"Does the size of a penis tell you how much of a man a guy is?"

He doesn't look embarrassed at all. "Well, son, I admire your frankness. You've come to the right man for the answer. Let's face it, in this job I see a lot of penises. Animal penises, that is. I can tell you one thing about those animals that you couldn't say about humans. They never worry about the size of the darn thing. One's as good as another—just like noses." At this he starts to chuckle. Then he leans on his broom and says, "Does that answer your question?"

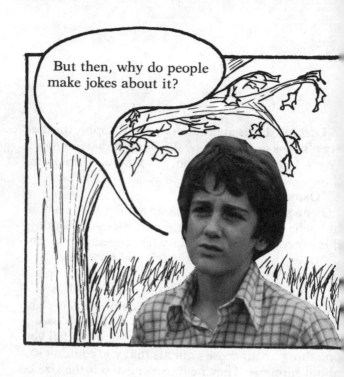

The zookeeper has an answer for this one too. "You know, people are funny. Sometimes they try to make other folks feel small, so they can feel big inside. Heck, the fact is—being big, or having big feet, or big anything—just has nothing to do with what kind of man you are." He smiles. "Any other questions, son?"

"No," I tell him. "That's about it. Thanks a lot."

"Glad I could help." And he goes back to his sweeping, whistling a little tune to himself.

I walk around for a while going over what the zookeeper said about people who make other people feel small so they can feel big inside. I decide that even though Tony's a pretty cool guy he probably feels just as confused inside as I do when it comes to sex and stuff.

Figuring this out makes me feel better, and I look around for my two best friends.

I find them sitting on a bench watching the penguins flapping in and out of the water.

Before I even sit down, Barry's asking me, "Where've you been? We were looking all over for you."

"I've been learning things," I tell him.

"What kinda things?"

I glance at Tony. "About my body." I take a deep breath. "About the penis."

Tony slaps his knee and starts up with his snorty laugh. "About your *what?* Can you believe this?" He turns to Barry, then back to me. "What has gotten into you, Jimmy? You used to be one cool guy, you know. I mean, I can dig wantin' to know about girls and stuff—but your *own* body? That's weird, man. Who wants to know about that?"

Barry says, "*I* do," and asks me, "What did you learn?" (I told you Barry was smart.)

So Barry wants to know what I learned and Tony thinks I'm weird. Well, Tony's attitude doesn't bother me as much as it used to. I figure he acts tough to make himself feel tough.

Since we spend so much time joking about sex and saying silly stuff, it seems like I should be able to say some of the true stuff that I found out.

Barry nudges me. "Come on, tell me what you learned."

I toss some popcorn to the pigeons, take a deep breath, stand up, and face the guys.

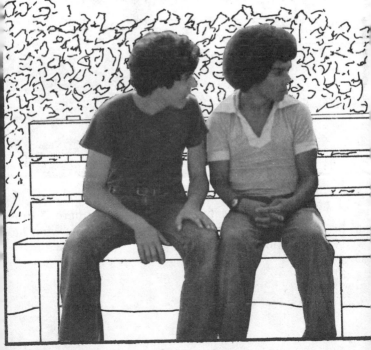

"Look, guys, it's like this. I thought I was a pretty cool guy and all, but then my body started acting crazy on me. I had a hunch it had to do with sex and stuff like that. But how could I still be cool on the outside when on the inside I didn't even know if I was normal or anything?

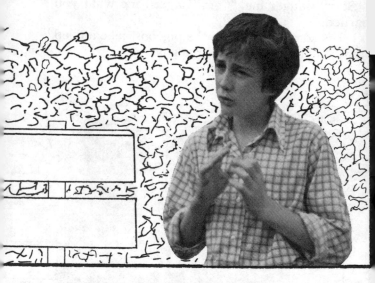

"And I knew if I asked Tony over here if those things ever happened to him, he'd do just what he's doing now. He'd laugh.

"So I had to find out for myself if these things were normal."

By now I'm pacing back and forth; I'm really into it.

I continue. "Well, when I was talking to Susie in the hall at school I got an erection, and we hadn't even touched. Turns out it's normal."

Tony pretends he isn't listening, but I know he is, and I dare him with a look to tell me what I'm saying isn't true.

"Then after you made those cracks about masturbation, I looked that up. And it turns out that if you do it or you don't, it's normal. There's just no way it can hurt you.

"Then I had this wet dream, and *that* was normal too.

"And now today, Tony here is giving me a hard time about penis size making a difference, and it just isn't true.

"As a matter of fact, a lot of things you hear about sex aren't true. The right people can tell you. You just have to ask the right people the right questions. That's what I did. I asked. And boy am I glad. Because now I feel normal again."

I can't believe I said all that. It's like once I got started it just kept coming out.

Barry was so fascinated he didn't close his mouth the whole time I was talking.

I look down at my feet because I figure Tony's about to give me a hard time and I don't know how I'll handle it.

Then I hear clapping—applause. I turn around. There's this whole bunch of people and they're clapping...*for me*. Kids and *grown-ups*. They must have been listening the whole time. I was so involved in putting things straight and feeling angry at Tony I didn't even notice them. Now I'm speechless.

A man comes over to shake my hand. "Proud to know you, son. I wish I had asked those questions when I was a boy."

A woman behind him comes toward me. "That was terrific. Where did you learn all that?"

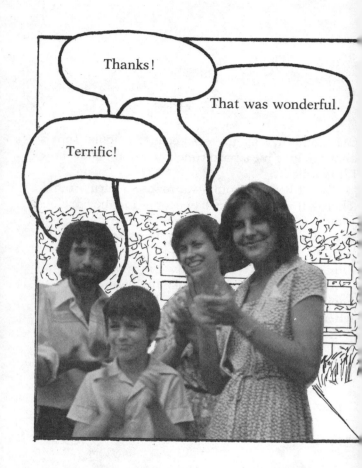

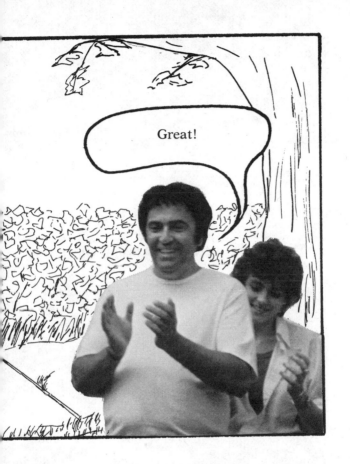

73

This is amazing. All these people congratulating *me!*

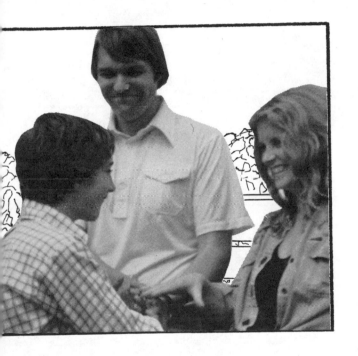

And wouldn't you know it, Tony's right there behind me shaking hands and introducing himself.

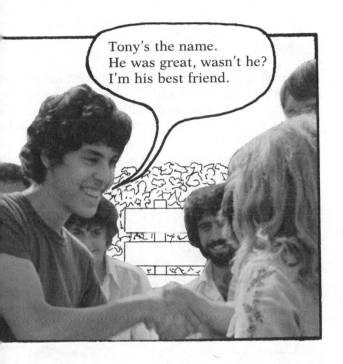

He turns to me and puts his arm around my shoulder. "Nice going, buddy."

Standing there with all these people smiling at me and shaking my hand, I decide it's normal to be confused about sex, especially when you're growing up. Talking honestly about sex seems to be an okay thing to do.

I turn around to see what Barry's been doing while Tony and I are enjoying all this glory. I find him without any trouble. He's right behind me talking to *Susie!*

I'm shocked.

I'm stunned.

I'm very surprised.

I'm *embarrassed.*

I can't ignore her, so I go over.

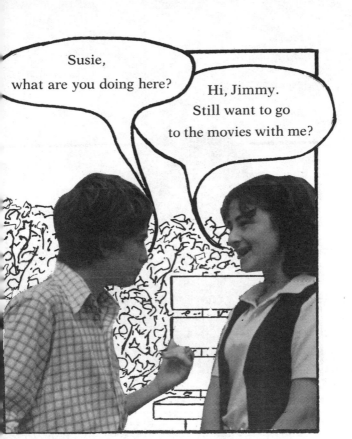

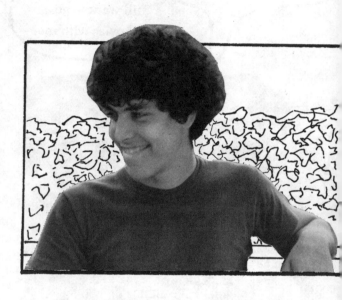

Tony gives me an "ooh-la-la" look, meaning, *Here's your big chance to be alone with a girl.*

But that's not what I want or how I feel.

Then I get an idea. "Sure, Susie," I say. "What if we all go together?"

Tony, Barry, and Susie's friend Teri think that's a terrific idea. I'm batting a thousand!

We pool our money, and it works out that if I can get in for under twelve this one more time, we have enough money for popcorn too.

All five of us have a real good time walking to the movies together.

This girl-boy thing isn't so bad, particularly when you're the hero of the day and you're feeling perfectly normal.

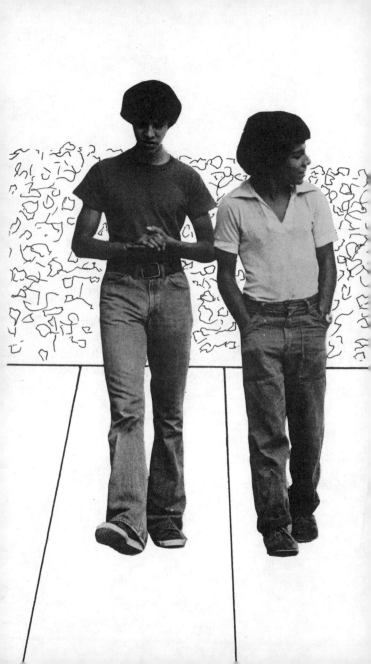

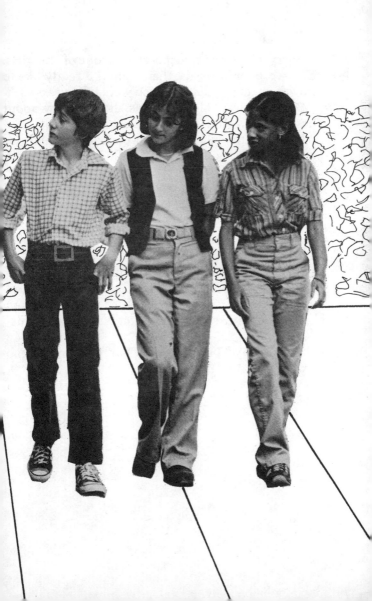

Barry mentions my speech in front of the girls. "You were terrific back there, Jim. I'd really like to know more about that stuff you were talking about."

Susie agrees! "Me too. Girls should know about these things." And Teri agrees with her.

I guess if the girls aren't embarrassed I might as well stay cool. So I say, real confident, "Sure, guys, any time."

That just leaves Tony. "Tony," I say, "do you want to hear more about this stuff?"

He sticks his hands in his pockets to give himself that real nonchalant look.

"I know all about that stuff," Tony says.

Barry and I look at each other. Good old Tony!

"But I got this little brother, see—uh—he doesn't know anything. You could talk to him. I'll listen in—just to make sure you don't make any mistakes."

"Sure, Tony," I say, smiling. Barry's grinning too as we all go into the theater.

By the way, I couldn't get into the movie for the kids' price. I guess there are some disadvantages to this growing-up business.

JEANNE BETANCOURT has taught junior high and high school, designed and taught courses in film and television, and run film programming workshops for librarians and educators. She is a contributing editor of *Channels* magazine, and is on the board of advisors of the Media Center for Children. Her published work includes articles and reviews and non-fiction for young readers. She currently lives with her daughter and her husband in New York City, where she is at work on a novel called THE RAINBOW KID.

DEBRA FRANCO and DAVID SHEPARD are a filmmaking/writing team based in New York. Ms. Franco is vice-president of New Day Films, a distribution cooperative of award-winning filmmakers. Mr. Shepard is a former film editor for public television and is the co-author of several screenplays. They are currently working on a feature film about adolescence.